THIS BOOK BELONGS TO:

CONTACT INFORMATION	
NAME:	
ADDRESS:	
PHONE:	

START / END DATES

_____ / _____ / _____   TO   _____ / _____ / _____

DEDICATION

This My Quotable Patients Journal is dedicated to all the nurses out there who want to monitor & record their patients' sayings and document their findings in the process.

You are my inspiration for producing books and I'm honored to be a part of keeping all of your patients saying notes and records organized.

This journal notebook will help you record the details of your patient's memorable quotes.

Thoughtfully put together with these sections to record: When was it said, Where, The Quote, & How would you describe it?

HOW TO USE THIS BOOK

The purpose of this book is to keep all of your Quotable Patient saying notes all in one place. It will help keep you organized.

This My Quotable Patients Journal will allow you to accurately document every detail about the funny things your patients say.

Here are examples of the prompts for you to fill in and write about your experience in this book:

1. When Was It Said - Write when the quote was said.

2. Where - Log where the quote was said & what setting.

3. The Quote - Blank lined notes to record what the quote was and who said it.

4. How Would You Describe It - In what situation was is said, funny, sincere, silly, quirky, creative, or weird.

NURSE/PATIENTS SAY

WHEN WAS IT SAID?	
WHERE?	

"

"

HOW WOULD YOU DESCRIBE IT?						AGE
☐ FUNNY	☐ SINCERE	☐ SILLY	☐ QUIRKY	☐ CREATIVE	☐ WEIRD	

NURSE/PATIENTS SAY

WHEN WAS IT SAID?	
WHERE?	

"

"

HOW WOULD YOU DESCRIBE IT?						AGE
☐ FUNNY	☐ SINCERE	☐ SILLY	☐ QUIRKY	☐ CREATIVE	☐ WEIRD	

NURSE/PATIENTS SAY

WHEN WAS IT SAID?	
WHERE?	

"

"

HOW WOULD YOU DESCRIBE IT?						AGE
☐ FUNNY	☐ SINCERE	☐ SILLY	☐ QUIRKY	☐ CREATIVE	☐ WEIRD	

NURSE/PATIENTS SAY

WHEN WAS IT SAID?	
WHERE?	

"

"

HOW WOULD YOU DESCRIBE IT?						AGE
□ FUNNY	□ SINCERE	□ SILLY	□ QUIRKY	□ CREATIVE	□ WEIRD	

NURSE/PATIENTS SAY

WHEN WAS IT SAID?	
WHERE?	

"

"

HOW WOULD YOU DESCRIBE IT?						AGE
□ FUNNY	□ SINCERE	□ SILLY	□ QUIRKY	□ CREATIVE	□ WEIRD	

NURSE/PATIENTS SAY

WHEN WAS IT SAID?	
WHERE?	

"

"

HOW WOULD YOU DESCRIBE IT?						AGE
□ FUNNY	□ SINCERE	□ SILLY	□ QUIRKY	□ CREATIVE	□ WEIRD	

NURSE/PATIENTS SAY

WHEN WAS IT SAID?	
WHERE?	

"

"

HOW WOULD YOU DESCRIBE IT?						AGE
□ FUNNY	□ SINCERE	□ SILLY	□ QUIRKY	□ CREATIVE	□ WEIRD	

NURSE/PATIENTS SAY

WHEN WAS IT SAID?	
WHERE?	

"

"

HOW WOULD YOU DESCRIBE IT?						AGE
☐ FUNNY	☐ SINCERE	☐ SILLY	☐ QUIRKY	☐ CREATIVE	☐ WEIRD	

NURSE/PATIENTS SAY

WHEN WAS IT SAID?	
WHERE?	

"

"

HOW WOULD YOU DESCRIBE IT?						AGE
☐ FUNNY	☐ SINCERE	☐ SILLY	☐ QUIRKY	☐ CREATIVE	☐ WEIRD	

NURSE/PATIENTS SAY

WHEN WAS IT SAID?	
WHERE?	

"

"

HOW WOULD YOU DESCRIBE IT?						AGE
□ FUNNY	□ SINCERE	□ SILLY	□ QUIRKY	□ CREATIVE	□ WEIRD	

NURSE/PATIENTS SAY

WHEN WAS IT SAID?	
WHERE?	

"

"

HOW WOULD YOU DESCRIBE IT?						AGE
□ FUNNY	□ SINCERE	□ SILLY	□ QUIRKY	□ CREATIVE	□ WEIRD	

NURSE/PATIENTS SAY

WHEN WAS IT SAID?	
WHERE?	

"

"

HOW WOULD YOU DESCRIBE IT?						AGE
□ FUNNY	□ SINCERE	□ SILLY	□ QUIRKY	□ CREATIVE	□ WEIRD	

NURSE/PATIENTS SAY

WHEN WAS IT SAID?	
WHERE?	

"

"

HOW WOULD YOU DESCRIBE IT?						AGE
□ FUNNY	□ SINCERE	□ SILLY	□ QUIRKY	□ CREATIVE	□ WEIRD	

NURSE/PATIENTS SAY

WHEN WAS IT SAID?	
WHERE?	

"

"

HOW WOULD YOU DESCRIBE IT?						AGE
□ FUNNY	□ SINCERE	□ SILLY	□ QUIRKY	□ CREATIVE	□ WEIRD	

NURSE/PATIENTS SAY

WHEN WAS IT SAID?	
WHERE?	

"

"

NURSE/PATIENTS SAY

WHEN WAS IT SAID?	
WHERE?	

"

"

HOW WOULD YOU DESCRIBE IT?						AGE
□ FUNNY	□ SINCERE	□ SILLY	□ QUIRKY	□ CREATIVE	□ WEIRD	

NURSE/PATIENTS SAY

WHEN WAS IT SAID?	
WHERE?	

"

"

HOW WOULD YOU DESCRIBE IT?						AGE
☐ FUNNY	☐ SINCERE	☐ SILLY	☐ QUIRKY	☐ CREATIVE	☐ WEIRD	

NURSE/PATIENTS SAY

WHEN WAS IT SAID?	
WHERE?	

"

"

HOW WOULD YOU DESCRIBE IT?						AGE
☐ FUNNY	☐ SINCERE	☐ SILLY	☐ QUIRKY	☐ CREATIVE	☐ WEIRD	

NURSE/PATIENTS SAY

WHEN WAS IT SAID?	
WHERE?	

"

"

HOW WOULD YOU DESCRIBE IT?						AGE
□ FUNNY	□ SINCERE	□ SILLY	□ QUIRKY	□ CREATIVE	□ WEIRD	

NURSE/PATIENTS SAY

WHEN WAS IT SAID?	
WHERE?	

"

"

HOW WOULD YOU DESCRIBE IT?						AGE
☐ FUNNY	☐ SINCERE	☐ SILLY	☐ QUIRKY	☐ CREATIVE	☐ WEIRD	

NURSE/PATIENTS SAY

WHEN WAS IT SAID?	
WHERE?	

"

"

HOW WOULD YOU DESCRIBE IT?						AGE
☐ FUNNY	☐ SINCERE	☐ SILLY	☐ QUIRKY	☐ CREATIVE	☐ WEIRD	

NURSE/PATIENTS SAY

WHEN WAS IT SAID?	
WHERE?	

"

"

HOW WOULD YOU DESCRIBE IT?						AGE
☐ FUNNY	☐ SINCERE	☐ SILLY	☐ QUIRKY	☐ CREATIVE	☐ WEIRD	

NURSE/PATIENTS SAY

WHEN WAS IT SAID?	
WHERE?	

"

"

HOW WOULD YOU DESCRIBE IT?						AGE
□ FUNNY	□ SINCERE	□ SILLY	□ QUIRKY	□ CREATIVE	□ WEIRD	

NURSE/PATIENTS SAY

WHEN WAS IT SAID?	
WHERE?	

"

						AGE
HOW WOULD YOU DESCRIBE IT?						
☐ FUNNY	☐ SINCERE	☐ SILLY	☐ QUIRKY	☐ CREATIVE	☐ WEIRD	

NURSE/PATIENTS SAY

WHEN WAS IT SAID?	
WHERE?	

"

"

HOW WOULD YOU DESCRIBE IT?						AGE
☐ FUNNY	☐ SINCERE	☐ SILLY	☐ QUIRKY	☐ CREATIVE	☐ WEIRD	

NURSE/PATIENTS SAY

WHEN WAS IT SAID?	
WHERE?	

"

"

HOW WOULD YOU DESCRIBE IT?						AGE
□ FUNNY	□ SINCERE	□ SILLY	□ QUIRKY	□ CREATIVE	□ WEIRD	

NURSE/PATIENTS SAY

WHEN WAS IT SAID?	
WHERE?	

"

"

HOW WOULD YOU DESCRIBE IT?						AGE
□ FUNNY	□ SINCERE	□ SILLY	□ QUIRKY	□ CREATIVE	□ WEIRD	

NURSE/PATIENTS SAY

WHEN WAS IT SAID?	
WHERE?	

"

"

HOW WOULD YOU DESCRIBE IT?						AGE
☐ FUNNY	☐ SINCERE	☐ SILLY	☐ QUIRKY	☐ CREATIVE	☐ WEIRD	

NURSE/PATIENTS SAY

WHEN WAS IT SAID?	
WHERE?	

"

"

HOW WOULD YOU DESCRIBE IT?						AGE
□ FUNNY	□ SINCERE	□ SILLY	□ QUIRKY	□ CREATIVE	□ WEIRD	

NURSE/PATIENTS SAY

WHEN WAS IT SAID?	
WHERE?	

"

"

HOW WOULD YOU DESCRIBE IT?						AGE
☐ FUNNY	☐ SINCERE	☐ SILLY	☐ QUIRKY	☐ CREATIVE	☐ WEIRD	

NURSE/PATIENTS SAY

WHEN WAS IT SAID?	
WHERE?	

"

"

HOW WOULD YOU DESCRIBE IT?						AGE
☐ FUNNY	☐ SINCERE	☐ SILLY	☐ QUIRKY	☐ CREATIVE	☐ WEIRD	

NURSE/PATIENTS SAY

WHEN WAS IT SAID?	
WHERE?	

"

"

HOW WOULD YOU DESCRIBE IT?						AGE
□ FUNNY	□ SINCERE	□ SILLY	□ QUIRKY	□ CREATIVE	□ WEIRD	

NURSE/PATIENTS SAY

WHEN WAS IT SAID?	
WHERE?	

″

″

HOW WOULD YOU DESCRIBE IT?						AGE
□ FUNNY	□ SINCERE	□ SILLY	□ QUIRKY	□ CREATIVE	□ WEIRD	

NURSE/PATIENTS SAY

WHEN WAS IT SAID?	
WHERE?	

"

"

HOW WOULD YOU DESCRIBE IT?						AGE
□ FUNNY	□ SINCERE	□ SILLY	□ QUIRKY	□ CREATIVE	□ WEIRD	

NURSE/PATIENTS SAY

WHEN WAS IT SAID?	
WHERE?	

"

"

HOW WOULD YOU DESCRIBE IT?						AGE
☐ FUNNY	☐ SINCERE	☐ SILLY	☐ QUIRKY	☐ CREATIVE	☐ WEIRD	

NURSE/PATIENTS SAY

WHEN WAS IT SAID?	
WHERE?	

"

"

HOW WOULD YOU DESCRIBE IT?						AGE
□ FUNNY	□ SINCERE	□ SILLY	□ QUIRKY	□ CREATIVE	□ WEIRD	

NURSE/PATIENTS SAY

WHEN WAS IT SAID?	
WHERE?	

"

"

HOW WOULD YOU DESCRIBE IT?						AGE
□ FUNNY	□ SINCERE	□ SILLY	□ QUIRKY	□ CREATIVE	□ WEIRD	

NURSE/PATIENTS SAY

WHEN WAS IT SAID?	
WHERE?	

"

"

HOW WOULD YOU DESCRIBE IT?						AGE
□ FUNNY	□ SINCERE	□ SILLY	□ QUIRKY	□ CREATIVE	□ WEIRD	

NURSE/PATIENTS SAY

WHEN WAS IT SAID?	
WHERE?	

"

"

HOW WOULD YOU DESCRIBE IT?						AGE
□ FUNNY	□ SINCERE	□ SILLY	□ QUIRKY	□ CREATIVE	□ WEIRD	

NURSE/PATIENTS SAY

WHEN WAS IT SAID?	
WHERE?	

″

_____

_____

_____

_____

_____

_____

_____

_____

_____

_____

_____

_____

_____

_____

″

HOW WOULD YOU DESCRIBE IT?						AGE
☐ FUNNY	☐ SINCERE	☐ SILLY	☐ QUIRKY	☐ CREATIVE	☐ WEIRD	

NURSE/PATIENTS SAY

WHEN WAS IT SAID?	
WHERE?	

"

"

NURSE/PATIENTS SAY

WHEN WAS IT SAID?	
WHERE?	

"

"

HOW WOULD YOU DESCRIBE IT?						AGE
☐ FUNNY	☐ SINCERE	☐ SILLY	☐ QUIRKY	☐ CREATIVE	☐ WEIRD	

NURSE/PATIENTS SAY

WHEN WAS IT SAID?	
WHERE?	

"

"

HOW WOULD YOU DESCRIBE IT?						AGE
□ FUNNY	□ SINCERE	□ SILLY	□ QUIRKY	□ CREATIVE	□ WEIRD	

NURSE/PATIENTS SAY

WHEN WAS IT SAID?	
WHERE?	

"

"

HOW WOULD YOU DESCRIBE IT?						AGE
☐ FUNNY	☐ SINCERE	☐ SILLY	☐ QUIRKY	☐ CREATIVE	☐ WEIRD	

NURSE/PATIENTS SAY

WHEN WAS IT SAID?	
WHERE?	

"

"

HOW WOULD YOU DESCRIBE IT?						AGE
☐ FUNNY	☐ SINCERE	☐ SILLY	☐ QUIRKY	☐ CREATIVE	☐ WEIRD	

NURSE/PATIENTS SAY

WHEN WAS IT SAID?	
WHERE?	

"

"

HOW WOULD YOU DESCRIBE IT?						AGE
☐ FUNNY	☐ SINCERE	☐ SILLY	☐ QUIRKY	☐ CREATIVE	☐ WEIRD	

NURSE/PATIENTS SAY

WHEN WAS IT SAID?	
WHERE?	

"

"

HOW WOULD YOU DESCRIBE IT?						AGE
☐ FUNNY	☐ SINCERE	☐ SILLY	☐ QUIRKY	☐ CREATIVE	☐ WEIRD	

NURSE/PATIENTS SAY

WHEN WAS IT SAID?	
WHERE?	

"

"

HOW WOULD YOU DESCRIBE IT?						AGE
☐ FUNNY	☐ SINCERE	☐ SILLY	☐ QUIRKY	☐ CREATIVE	☐ WEIRD	

NURSE/PATIENTS SAY

WHEN WAS IT SAID?	
WHERE?	

"

"

HOW WOULD YOU DESCRIBE IT?						AGE
☐ FUNNY	☐ SINCERE	☐ SILLY	☐ QUIRKY	☐ CREATIVE	☐ WEIRD	

NURSE/PATIENTS SAY

WHEN WAS IT SAID?	
WHERE?	

"

"

HOW WOULD YOU DESCRIBE IT?						AGE
☐ FUNNY	☐ SINCERE	☐ SILLY	☐ QUIRKY	☐ CREATIVE	☐ WEIRD	

NURSE/PATIENTS SAY

WHEN WAS IT SAID?	
WHERE?	

"

"

HOW WOULD YOU DESCRIBE IT?						AGE
□ FUNNY	□ SINCERE	□ SILLY	□ QUIRKY	□ CREATIVE	□ WEIRD	

NURSE/PATIENTS SAY

WHEN WAS IT SAID?	
WHERE?	

"

"

HOW WOULD YOU DESCRIBE IT?						AGE
☐ FUNNY	☐ SINCERE	☐ SILLY	☐ QUIRKY	☐ CREATIVE	☐ WEIRD	

NURSE/PATIENTS SAY

WHEN WAS IT SAID?	
WHERE?	

"

"

HOW WOULD YOU DESCRIBE IT?						AGE
☐ FUNNY	☐ SINCERE	☐ SILLY	☐ QUIRKY	☐ CREATIVE	☐ WEIRD	

NURSE/PATIENTS SAY

WHEN WAS IT SAID?	
WHERE?	

"

"

HOW WOULD YOU DESCRIBE IT?						AGE
☐ FUNNY	☐ SINCERE	☐ SILLY	☐ QUIRKY	☐ CREATIVE	☐ WEIRD	

NURSE/PATIENTS SAY

WHEN WAS IT SAID?	
WHERE?	

"

"

HOW WOULD YOU DESCRIBE IT?						AGE
☐ FUNNY	☐ SINCERE	☐ SILLY	☐ QUIRKY	☐ CREATIVE	☐ WEIRD	

NURSE/PATIENTS SAY

WHEN WAS IT SAID?	
WHERE?	

"

"

HOW WOULD YOU DESCRIBE IT?						AGE
☐ FUNNY	☐ SINCERE	☐ SILLY	☐ QUIRKY	☐ CREATIVE	☐ WEIRD	

NURSE/PATIENTS SAY

WHEN WAS IT SAID?	
WHERE?	

"

"

HOW WOULD YOU DESCRIBE IT?						AGE
□ FUNNY	□ SINCERE	□ SILLY	□ QUIRKY	□ CREATIVE	□ WEIRD	

NURSE/PATIENTS SAY

WHEN WAS IT SAID?	
WHERE?	

"

"

HOW WOULD YOU DESCRIBE IT?						AGE
□ FUNNY	□ SINCERE	□ SILLY	□ QUIRKY	□ CREATIVE	□ WEIRD	

NURSE/PATIENTS SAY

WHEN WAS IT SAID?	
WHERE?	

"

"

HOW WOULD YOU DESCRIBE IT?						AGE
☐ FUNNY	☐ SINCERE	☐ SILLY	☐ QUIRKY	☐ CREATIVE	☐ WEIRD	

NURSE/PATIENTS SAY

WHEN WAS IT SAID?	
WHERE?	

"

"

HOW WOULD YOU DESCRIBE IT?						AGE
☐ FUNNY	☐ SINCERE	☐ SILLY	☐ QUIRKY	☐ CREATIVE	☐ WEIRD	

NURSE/PATIENTS SAY

WHEN WAS IT SAID?	
WHERE?	

"

"

HOW WOULD YOU DESCRIBE IT?						AGE
□ FUNNY	□ SINCERE	□ SILLY	□ QUIRKY	□ CREATIVE	□ WEIRD	

NURSE/PATIENTS SAY

WHEN WAS IT SAID?	
WHERE?	

"

"

HOW WOULD YOU DESCRIBE IT?						AGE
☐ FUNNY	☐ SINCERE	☐ SILLY	☐ QUIRKY	☐ CREATIVE	☐ WEIRD	

NURSE/PATIENTS SAY

WHEN WAS IT SAID?	
WHERE?	

"

"

NURSE/PATIENTS SAY

WHEN WAS IT SAID?	
WHERE?	

"

"

HOW WOULD YOU DESCRIBE IT?						AGE
☐ FUNNY	☐ SINCERE	☐ SILLY	☐ QUIRKY	☐ CREATIVE	☐ WEIRD	

NURSE/PATIENTS SAY

WHEN WAS IT SAID?	
WHERE?	

"

"

HOW WOULD YOU DESCRIBE IT?						AGE
☐ FUNNY	☐ SINCERE	☐ SILLY	☐ QUIRKY	☐ CREATIVE	☐ WEIRD	

NURSE/PATIENTS SAY

WHEN WAS IT SAID?	
WHERE?	

"

"

HOW WOULD YOU DESCRIBE IT?						AGE
☐ FUNNY	☐ SINCERE	☐ SILLY	☐ QUIRKY	☐ CREATIVE	☐ WEIRD	

NURSE/PATIENTS SAY

WHEN WAS IT SAID?	
WHERE?	

"

"

HOW WOULD YOU DESCRIBE IT?						AGE
□ FUNNY	□ SINCERE	□ SILLY	□ QUIRKY	□ CREATIVE	□ WEIRD	

NURSE/PATIENTS SAY

WHEN WAS IT SAID?	
WHERE?	

"

"

NURSE/PATIENTS SAY

WHEN WAS IT SAID?	
WHERE?	

"

"

HOW WOULD YOU DESCRIBE IT?						AGE
□ FUNNY	□ SINCERE	□ SILLY	□ QUIRKY	□ CREATIVE	□ WEIRD	

NURSE/PATIENTS SAY

WHEN WAS IT SAID?	
WHERE?	

"

"

HOW WOULD YOU DESCRIBE IT?						AGE
☐ FUNNY	☐ SINCERE	☐ SILLY	☐ QUIRKY	☐ CREATIVE	☐ WEIRD	

NURSE/PATIENTS SAY

WHEN WAS IT SAID?	
WHERE?	

"

"

HOW WOULD YOU DESCRIBE IT?						AGE
☐ FUNNY	☐ SINCERE	☐ SILLY	☐ QUIRKY	☐ CREATIVE	☐ WEIRD	

NURSE/PATIENTS SAY

WHEN WAS IT SAID?	
WHERE?	

"

"

HOW WOULD YOU DESCRIBE IT?						AGE
☐ FUNNY	☐ SINCERE	☐ SILLY	☐ QUIRKY	☐ CREATIVE	☐ WEIRD	

NURSE/PATIENTS SAY

WHEN WAS IT SAID?	
WHERE?	

"

"

HOW WOULD YOU DESCRIBE IT?						AGE
☐ FUNNY	☐ SINCERE	☐ SILLY	☐ QUIRKY	☐ CREATIVE	☐ WEIRD	

NURSE/PATIENTS SAY

WHEN WAS IT SAID?	
WHERE?	

″

″

HOW WOULD YOU DESCRIBE IT?						AGE
□ FUNNY	□ SINCERE	□ SILLY	□ QUIRKY	□ CREATIVE	□ WEIRD	

NURSE/PATIENTS SAY

WHEN WAS IT SAID?	
WHERE?	

"

"

HOW WOULD YOU DESCRIBE IT?						AGE
☐ FUNNY	☐ SINCERE	☐ SILLY	☐ QUIRKY	☐ CREATIVE	☐ WEIRD	

NURSE/PATIENTS SAY

WHEN WAS IT SAID?	
WHERE?	

"

"

HOW WOULD YOU DESCRIBE IT?						AGE
☐ FUNNY	☐ SINCERE	☐ SILLY	☐ QUIRKY	☐ CREATIVE	☐ WEIRD	

NURSE/PATIENTS SAY

WHEN WAS IT SAID?	
WHERE?	

"

"

HOW WOULD YOU DESCRIBE IT?						AGE
☐ FUNNY	☐ SINCERE	☐ SILLY	☐ QUIRKY	☐ CREATIVE	☐ WEIRD	

NURSE/PATIENTS SAY

WHEN WAS IT SAID?	
WHERE?	

"

"

HOW WOULD YOU DESCRIBE IT?						AGE
☐ FUNNY	☐ SINCERE	☐ SILLY	☐ QUIRKY	☐ CREATIVE	☐ WEIRD	

NURSE/PATIENTS SAY

WHEN WAS IT SAID?	
WHERE?	

"

"

HOW WOULD YOU DESCRIBE IT?						AGE
□ FUNNY	□ SINCERE	□ SILLY	□ QUIRKY	□ CREATIVE	□ WEIRD	

NURSE/PATIENTS SAY

WHEN WAS IT SAID?	
WHERE?	

"

"

HOW WOULD YOU DESCRIBE IT?						AGE
☐ FUNNY	☐ SINCERE	☐ SILLY	☐ QUIRKY	☐ CREATIVE	☐ WEIRD	

NURSE/PATIENTS SAY

WHEN WAS IT SAID?	
WHERE?	

"

"

HOW WOULD YOU DESCRIBE IT?						AGE
□ FUNNY	□ SINCERE	□ SILLY	□ QUIRKY	□ CREATIVE	□ WEIRD	

NURSE/PATIENTS SAY

WHEN WAS IT SAID?	
WHERE?	

"

"

HOW WOULD YOU DESCRIBE IT?						AGE
□ FUNNY	□ SINCERE	□ SILLY	□ QUIRKY	□ CREATIVE	□ WEIRD	

NURSE/PATIENTS SAY

WHEN WAS IT SAID?	
WHERE?	

"

"

HOW WOULD YOU DESCRIBE IT?						AGE
□ FUNNY	□ SINCERE	□ SILLY	□ QUIRKY	□ CREATIVE	□ WEIRD	

NURSE/PATIENTS SAY

WHEN WAS IT SAID?	
WHERE?	

"

"

HOW WOULD YOU DESCRIBE IT?						AGE
☐ FUNNY	☐ SINCERE	☐ SILLY	☐ QUIRKY	☐ CREATIVE	☐ WEIRD	

NURSE/PATIENTS SAY

WHEN WAS IT SAID?	
WHERE?	

"

"

HOW WOULD YOU DESCRIBE IT?						AGE
☐ FUNNY	☐ SINCERE	☐ SILLY	☐ QUIRKY	☐ CREATIVE	☐ WEIRD	

NURSE/PATIENTS SAY

WHEN WAS IT SAID?	
WHERE?	

"

"

HOW WOULD YOU DESCRIBE IT?						AGE
☐ FUNNY	☐ SINCERE	☐ SILLY	☐ QUIRKY	☐ CREATIVE	☐ WEIRD	

NURSE/PATIENTS SAY

WHEN WAS IT SAID?	
WHERE?	

"

"

HOW WOULD YOU DESCRIBE IT?						AGE
□ FUNNY	□ SINCERE	□ SILLY	□ QUIRKY	□ CREATIVE	□ WEIRD	

NURSE/PATIENTS SAY

WHEN WAS IT SAID?	
WHERE?	

"

"

HOW WOULD YOU DESCRIBE IT?						AGE
☐ FUNNY	☐ SINCERE	☐ SILLY	☐ QUIRKY	☐ CREATIVE	☐ WEIRD	

NURSE/PATIENTS SAY

WHEN WAS IT SAID?	
WHERE?	

"

"

HOW WOULD YOU DESCRIBE IT?						AGE
□ FUNNY	□ SINCERE	□ SILLY	□ QUIRKY	□ CREATIVE	□ WEIRD	

NURSE/PATIENTS SAY

WHEN WAS IT SAID?	
WHERE?	

"

"

HOW WOULD YOU DESCRIBE IT?						AGE
☐ FUNNY	☐ SINCERE	☐ SILLY	☐ QUIRKY	☐ CREATIVE	☐ WEIRD	

NURSE/PATIENTS SAY

WHEN WAS IT SAID?	
WHERE?	

"

"

HOW WOULD YOU DESCRIBE IT?						AGE
☐ FUNNY	☐ SINCERE	☐ SILLY	☐ QUIRKY	☐ CREATIVE	☐ WEIRD	

NURSE/PATIENTS SAY

WHEN WAS IT SAID?	
WHERE?	

"

"

HOW WOULD YOU DESCRIBE IT?						AGE
☐ FUNNY	☐ SINCERE	☐ SILLY	☐ QUIRKY	☐ CREATIVE	☐ WEIRD	

NURSE/PATIENTS SAY

WHEN WAS IT SAID?	
WHERE?	

"

"

HOW WOULD YOU DESCRIBE IT?						AGE
☐ FUNNY	☐ SINCERE	☐ SILLY	☐ QUIRKY	☐ CREATIVE	☐ WEIRD	

NURSE/PATIENTS SAY

WHEN WAS IT SAID?	
WHERE?	

"

"

HOW WOULD YOU DESCRIBE IT?						AGE
☐ FUNNY	☐ SINCERE	☐ SILLY	☐ QUIRKY	☐ CREATIVE	☐ WEIRD	

NURSE/PATIENTS SAY

WHEN WAS IT SAID?	
WHERE?	

"

"

HOW WOULD YOU DESCRIBE IT?						AGE
☐ FUNNY	☐ SINCERE	☐ SILLY	☐ QUIRKY	☐ CREATIVE	☐ WEIRD	

NURSE/PATIENTS SAY

WHEN WAS IT SAID?	
WHERE?	

"

"

HOW WOULD YOU DESCRIBE IT?						AGE
☐ FUNNY	☐ SINCERE	☐ SILLY	☐ QUIRKY	☐ CREATIVE	☐ WEIRD	

NURSE/PATIENTS SAY

WHEN WAS IT SAID?	
WHERE?	

"

"

HOW WOULD YOU DESCRIBE IT?						AGE
□ FUNNY	□ SINCERE	□ SILLY	□ QUIRKY	□ CREATIVE	□ WEIRD	